I0790304

INTRODUCTION

The Autoimmune Paleo Diet

The Autoimmune Paleo (AIP) diet is derived from the Paleolithic diet.

The Paleolithic diet, known today as the modern Paleo diet, originated from the ideas of a gastroenterologist in 1975, Dr. Walter Voegtlin. Later in 1985, Dr. Boyd Eaton wrote a scientific paper about Paleolithic nutrition, published in the New England Journal of Medicine. However, the diet has been made popular by Dr. Loren Cordain, founder of the Paleo Movement, in 2002.

The Autoimmune Protocol (AIP) is a diet that aims to reduce inflammation, pain, and other symptoms caused by autoimmune diseases, such as lupus, inflammatory bowel disease (IBD), celiac disease, and rheumatoid arthritis (1Trusted Source).

Many people who have followed the AIP diet report improvements in the way they feel, as well as reductions in common symptoms of autoimmune disorders, such as fatigue and gut or joint pain. Yet, while research on this diet is promising, it's also limited.

This book offers a comprehensive overview of the AIP diet, including the science behind it, as well as what is currently known about its ability to reduce symptoms of autoimmune disorders

Gut Inflammation Relief

The AIP diet is an elimination and reintroduction protocol which aims to reduce inflammation in the gut, heal the gastrointestinal tract and in turn, reduce overall systemic inflammation. It is a diet targeted specifically at autoimmune diseases.

Traits Of The Aip Diet

The AIP diet focuses on removing foods from the diet that people are commonly sensitive to, in order to lower overall inflammation.

The AIP diet is a version of the original Paleo diet which addresses underlying inflammation stemming from the gut, and can be a major driver of autoimmune disease. The AIP diet aims to bring the gut microbiota back into balance, whilst optimizing overall nutrient intake.

Beyond the Traditional Paleo Diet for Autoimmune Conditions

The traditional Paleo diet eliminates all grains and processed foods. It focuses on whole, nutrient-dense foods, such as fruit and vegetables, organic meats, eggs, and wild-caught fish. However, this is often not comprehensive enough for chronic autoimmune diseases, as not enough of the immune triggers are removed.

Because the AIP diet is utilized specifically for autoimmune diseases, it is almost always necessary to employ additional modalities to treat the condition. Herbal and nutritional medicines may be prescribed alongside an autoimmune diet as a part of a protocol to treat you as a whole person, rather than just targeting the disease process in isolation.

Not everyone must strictly avoid all the eliminated foods from the diet permanently, as not everyone with an autoimmune disease is sensitive to these foods.

The Gut And Immunity

Probiotics and Digestive System MicrobiomeThere is a complex symbiotic relationship between the immune system of the host (person) and the gut microbiota.

The microbiota is the population of the microbes which reside in the gut. It carries out digestion and fermentation of carbohydrates, synthesizes certain vitamins, provides development of the gut-associated lymphoid tissue (GALT), and also prevents the colonization of pathogens. The host will provide nutrients for the survival of the bacteria.

Your Microbiota and Your Microbiome

Let's take a quick look at these increasingly common terms...

The human microbiota comprises the populations of microbial species that live on or in the human body – the bacteria, viruses and fungi that call our bodies home.

It is estimated that each of us has anywhere between 10 trillion and 100 trillion microbial cells in a symbiotic relationship. These make up the human microbiota.

All of the genes inside these microbial cells, meanwhile, are what constitute the microbiome.

Watch this video to understand more about your body's ecosystem (produced by the Genetic Science Learning Center)

Disturbance Of The Gut Microbiome

When there is disturbance to this symbiotic relationship due to poor dietary or lifestyle choices, medications such as antibiotics, and/or stress, the microbiota could potentially contribute towards the development of certain infectious disease or trigger an autoimmune process.

The AIP diet has a strong emphasis on reducing inflammation in the gut as the digestive system plays a major role in the overall function of the immune system. Eliminating foods that reduce inflammation is important, as foods which irritate the gut can potentially exacerbate autoimmunity.

What Conditions May Benefit From The Aip Diet?

Many autoimmune conditions may benefit from the AIP diet, including:

Hashimoto's Disease

Rheumatoid Arthritis

Coeliac Disease

Adrenal fatigue

Recurrent viral infections or low immunity

Poly Cystic Ovarian Syndrome (PCOS)

Multiple Sclerosis

Sjogren's

Type 1 Diabetes

Lupus (SLE)

Other factors to consider with the AIP

As autoimmune conditions can potentially be very complex, there are many other factors that need to be taken into consideration in addition to addressing diet when dealing with conditions like the aforementioned.

Hormonal imbalances, and the hypothalamic-pituitary-adrenal/ovarian axis need to be assessed and addressed. Potential infections, either acute or chronic also need to be dealt with. Digestive bacterial imbalances, such as Small Intestinal Bacterial Overgrowth (SIBO), or even parasitic infections, should be rectified. Blood sugar issues such as insulin resistance, or pre-diabetes need to also be identified.

Other factors such as your sensitivity to high FODMAPs foods (fermentable oligosaccharides, disaccharides, monosaccharides and polyols), and your tolerance to histamines and salicylates needs to be assessed individually in order to tailor an autoimmune protocol that is suitable for you.

There may also be specific testing that needs to be conducted in order to monitor disease progression or improvement whilst endeavoring to treat autoimmune diseases. These may include, but are not limited to inflammatory markers, specific hormones, blood glucose testing, imaging scans, and specimen cultures.

What can be eaten and what is excluded with AIP?

The table below outlines what should be eaten and excluded during the elimination phase of the AIP diet:

Included with AIP

Excluded from AIP

All vegetables except nightshades

Fresh fruit

Coconut (oil, milk, flour, and coconut aminos)

Fermented food (kefir, kombucha, coconut yoghurt, Kim chi, sauerkraut)

Organic grass fed meat, organ meat, poultry

Seafood

Herbal teas

Vinegar

Oils and fats (olive oil, ghee, lard, avocado oil)

Herbs (ginger, turmeric, basil, thyme, sage, oregano, rosemary, mint, cinnamon)

Gelatin

Arrowroot starch

Nuts

Seeds

Beans and legumes

Grains

Dairy products

Dried fruit

All processed foods

Eggs

Chocolate

Nightshade plants (tomato, potato, capsicum, eggplant, chilli)

Seed herbs (mustard seeds, coriander seeds, fennel, fenugreek)

Tapioca

Vegetable oils

Artificial sweeteners

Stevia, xylitol

High FODMAPs food such as fruit (onion, coconut, nectarines) may bother some people and these need to be eliminated during the first phase. Re-introduction of high FODMAPs foods should be done with care, you can read more about how to reintroduce these foods

How To Implement The Aip Diet:

It is recommended to follow the elimination diet for at least 30 days, and up to 90 days. Beginning the elimination phase can be done cold turkey, or one category of food can be removed at a time, for a week. E.g. Grains are removed the first week, followed by dairy products the second week, nightshades the third week, eggs the fourth week and so on.

When positive change is observed, the reintroduction phase is commenced. This needs to be done slowly and systematically, to reduce the chances of a reaction. Reactions may not always occur immediately, there may be slow increases of symptoms that may not be noticed as easily.

Choose a food group that is important to you, and start with that group. If dairy is chosen, choose a food like ghee with a low amount of milk proteins, followed by butter, cream, yoghurt, cheese and milk.

Eggs should be reintroduced with yolks only first. Nightshades should be reintroduced individually (potatoes, tomatoes, eggplants).

Only introduce one food at a time and allow for three full days between foods to observe any potential reactions to that food before moving on to the next. If a food has been eaten for three days without any autoimmune symptoms, it can be assumed that that food is safe for you.

One Day On The Aip Diet:

Below are examples of meals that you could eat on the AIP diet:

Breakfast

Lunch

Dinner

Snacks

Organic bacon
Sweet potato
Sautéed kale, and zucchini
Chicken and ginger stir-fry
Cauliflower rice

What Is The Autoimmune Protocol Diet?

A healthy immune system is designed to produce antibodies that attack foreign or harmful cells in your body.

However, in people with autoimmune disorders, the immune system tends to produce antibodies that, rather than fight infections, attack healthy cells and tissues.

This can result in a range of symptoms, including joint pain, fatigue, abdominal pain, diarrhea, brain fog, and tissue and nerve damage.

A few examples of autoimmune disorders include rheumatoid arthritis, lupus, IBD, type 1 diabetes, and psoriasis.

Autoimmune diseases are thought to be caused by a variety of factors, including genetic propensity, infection, stress, inflammation, and medication use.

Also, some research suggests that, in susceptible individuals, damage to the gut barrier can lead to increased intestinal permeability, also known as "leaky gut," which may trigger the development of certain autoimmune diseases (2).

Certain foods are believed to possibly increase the gut's permeability, thereby increasing your likelihood of leaky gut.

The AIP diet focuses on eliminating these foods and replacing them with health-promoting, nutrient-dense foods that are thought to help heal the gut, and ultimately, reduce inflammation and symptoms of autoimmune diseases (3).

It also removes certain ingredients like gluten, which may cause abnormal immune responses in susceptible individuals (4, 5).

While experts believe that a leaky gut may be a plausible explanation for the inflammation experienced by people with autoimmune disorders, they warn that the current research makes it impossible to confirm a cause-and-effect relationship between the two (2).

How Does It Work?

The AIP diet resembles the paleo diet, both in the types of foods allowed and avoided, as well as in the phases that comprise it. Due to their similarities, many consider the AIP diet an extension of the paleo diet — though AIP may be seen as a stricter version of it.

The AIP diet consists of two main phases.

The Elimination Phase

The first phase is an elimination phase that involves the removal of foods and medications believed to cause gut inflammation, imbalances between levels of good and bad bacteria in the gut, or an immune response (1, 3).

During this phase, foods like grains, legumes, nuts, seeds, nightshade vegetables, eggs, and dairy are completely avoided.

Tobacco, alcohol, coffee, oils, food additives, refined and processed sugars, and certain medications, such as non-steroidal anti-inflammatory drugs (NSAIDs) should also be avoided (1).

Examples of NSAIDs include ibuprofen, naproxen, diclofenac, and high dose aspirin.

On the other hand, this phase encourages the consumption of fresh, nutrient-dense foods, minimally processed meat, fermented foods, and bone broth. It also emphasizes the improvement of lifestyle factors, such as stress, sleep, and physical activity (1).

The length of the elimination phase of the diet varies, as it's typically maintained until a person feels a noticeable reduction in symptoms. On average, most people maintain this phase for 30–90 days, but some may notice improvements as early as within the first 3 weeks (1, 6).

The Reintroduction Phase

Once a measurable improvement in symptoms and overall well-being occurs, the reintroduction phase can begin. During this phase, the avoided foods are gradually reintroduced into the diet, one at a time, based on the person's tolerance.

The goal of this phase is to identify which foods contribute to a person's symptoms and reintroduce all foods that don't cause any symptoms while continuing to avoid those that do. This allows for the widest dietary variety a person can tolerate.

During this phase, foods should be reintroduced one at a time, allowing for a period of 5–7 days before reintroducing a different food. This allows a person enough time to notice if any of their symptoms reappear before continuing the reintroduction process (1).

Foods that are well tolerated can be added back into the diet, while those that trigger symptoms should continue to be avoided. Keep in mind that your food tolerance may change over time.

As such, you may want to repeat the reintroduction test for foods that initially failed the test every once in a while.

Step-By-Step Reintroduction Protocol

Here's a step-by-step approach to reintroducing foods that were avoided during the elimination phase of the AIP diet.

Step 1. Choose one food to reintroduce. Plan to consume this food a few times per day on the testing day, then avoid it completely for 5–6 days.

Step 2. Eat a small amount, such as 1 teaspoon of the food, and wait 15 minutes to see if you have a reaction.

Step 3. If you experience any symptoms, end the test and avoid this food. If you have no symptoms, eat a slightly larger portion, such as 1 1/2 tablespoons, of the same food and monitor how you feel for 2–3 hours.

Step 4. If you experience any symptoms over this period, end the test and avoid this food. If no symptoms occur, eat a normal portion of the same food and avoid it for 5–6 days without reintroducing any other foods.

Step 5. If you experience no symptoms for 5–6 days, you may reincorporate the tested food into your diet, and repeat this 5-step reintroduction process with a new food.

It's best to avoid reintroducing foods under circumstances that tend to increase inflammation and make it difficult to interpret results. These include during an infection, following a poor night's sleep, when feeling unusually stressed, or following a strenuous workout.

Additionally, it's sometimes recommended to reintroduce foods in a particular order. For example, when reintroducing dairy, choose dairy products with the lowest lactose concentration to reintroduce first, such as ghee or fermented dairy products.

Foods To Eat And Avoid

The AIP diet has strict recommendations regarding which foods to eat or avoid during its elimination phase (7, 8).

Foods To Avoid

Grains: rice, wheat, oats, barley, rye, etc., as well as foods derived from them, such as pasta, bread, and breakfast cereals

Legumes: lentils, beans, peas, peanuts, etc., as well as foods derived from them, such as tofu, tempeh, mock meats, or peanut butter

Nightshade vegetables: eggplants, peppers, potatoes, tomatoes, tomatillos, etc., as well as spices derived from nightshade vegetables, such as paprika

Eggs: whole eggs, egg whites, or foods containing these ingredients

Dairy: cow's, goat's, or sheep's milk, as well as foods derived from these milks, such as cream, cheese, butter, or ghee; dairy-based protein powders or other supplements should also be avoided

Nuts and seeds: all nuts and seeds and foods derived from them, such as flours, butter, or oils; also includes cocoa and seed-based spices, such as coriander, cumin, anise, fennel, fenugreek, mustard, and nutmeg

Certain beverages: alcohol and coffee

Processed vegetable oils: canola, rapeseed, corn, cottonseed, palm kernel, safflower, soybean, or sunflower oils

Refined or processed sugars: cane or beet sugar, corn syrup, brown rice syrup, and barley malt syrup; also includes sweets, soda, candy, frozen desserts, and chocolate, which may contain these ingredients

Food additives and artificial sweeteners: trans fats, food colorings, emulsifiers, and thickeners, as well as artificial sweeteners, such as stevia, mannitol, and xylitol

Some AIP protocols further recommend avoiding all fruit — both fresh or dried — during the elimination phase. Others allow the inclusion of 10–40 grams of fructose per day, which amounts to around 1–2 portions of fruit per day.

Although not specified in all AIP protocols, some also suggest avoiding algae, such as spirulina or chlorella, during the elimination phase, as this type of sea vegetable may also stimulate an immune response (9).

Foods To Eat

Vegetables: a variety of vegetables except for nightshade vegetables and algae, which should be avoided

Fresh fruit: a variety of fresh fruit, in moderation

Tubers: sweet potatoes, taro, yams, as well as Jerusalem or Chinese artichokes

Minimally processed meat: wild game, fish, seafood, organ meat, and poultry; meats should be wild, grass-fed or pasture-raised, whenever possible

Fermented, probiotic-rich foods: nondairy-based fermented food, such as kombucha, kimchi, sauerkraut, pickles, and coconut kefir; probiotic supplements may also be consumed

Minimally processed vegetable oils: olive oil, avocado oil, or coconut oil

Herbs and spices: as long as they're not derived from a seed

Vinegars: balsamic, apple cider, and red wine vinegar, as long as they're free of added sugars

Natural sweeteners: maple syrup and honey, in moderation

Certain teas: green and black tea at average intakes of up to 3–4 cups per day

Bone broth

Despite being allowed, some protocols further recommend that you moderate your intake of salt, saturated and omega-6 fats, natural sugars, such as honey or maple syrup, as well as coconut-based foods.

Depending on the AIP protocol at hand, small amounts of fruit may also be allowed. This usually amounts to a maximum intake of 10–40 grams of fructose per day, or the equivalent of about 1–2 portions of fresh fruit.

Some protocols further suggest moderating your intake of high glycemic fruits and vegetables, including dried fruit, sweet potatoes, and plantain.

The glycemic index (GI) is a system used to rank foods on a scale of 0 to 100, based on how much they will increase blood sugar levels, compared with white bread. High glycemic fruits and vegetables are those ranked 70 or above on the GI scale (10).

Summary

The AIP diet typically consists of minimally processed, nutrient-dense foods. The lists above specify which foods to eat or avoid during the elimination phase of the AIP diet.

Does The Aip Diet Work?

Though research on the AIP diet is limited, some evidence suggests that it may reduce inflammation and symptoms of certain autoimmune diseases.

May help heal a leaky gut

People with autoimmune diseases often have a leaky gut, and experts believe there may be a link between the inflammation they experience and the permeability of their gut (2, 3, 11, 12).

A healthy gut typically has a low permeability. This allows it to act as a good barrier and prevent food and waste remains from leaking into the bloodstream.

However, a highly permeable or leaky gut allows foreign particles to crossover into the bloodstream, in turn, possibly causing inflammation.

In parallel, there's growing evidence that the foods you eat can influence your gut's immunity and function, and in some cases, possibly even reduce the degree of inflammation you experience (13, 14).

One hypothesis entertained by researchers is that by helping heal leaky gut, the AIP diet may help reduce the degree of inflammation a person experiences.

Although scientific evidence is currently limited, a handful of studies suggests that the AIP diet may help reduce inflammation or symptoms caused by it, at least among a subset of people with certain autoimmune disorders (6, 7, 15).

However, more research is needed to specifically understand the exact ways in which the AIP diet may help, as well as the precise circumstances under which it may do so (2).

May reduce inflammation and symptoms of some autoimmune disorders

To date, the AIP diet has been tested in a small group of people and yielded seemingly positive results.

For instance, in a recent 11-week study in 15 people with IBD on an AIP diet, participants reported experiencing significantly fewer IBD-related symptoms by the end of the study. However, no significant changes in markers of inflammation were observed (15).

Similarly, a small study had people with IBD follow the AIP diet for 11 weeks. Participants reported significant improvements in bowel frequency, stress, and the ability to perform leisure or sport activities as early as 3 weeks into the study (6).

In another study, 16 women with Hashimoto's thyroiditis, an autoimmune disorder affecting the thyroid gland, followed the AIP diet for 10 weeks. By the end of the study, inflammation and disease-related symptoms decreased by 29% and 68%, respect-ively.

Participants also reported significant improvements in their quality of life, despite there being no significant differences in their measures of thyroid function (7).

Although promising, studies remain small and few. Also, to date, they have only been performed on a small subset of people with autoimmune disorders. Therefore, more research is needed before strong conclusions can be made.

Possible downsides

The AIP diet is considered an elimination diet, which makes it very restrictive and potentially hard to follow for some, especially in its elimination phase.

The elimination phase of this diet can also make it difficult for people to eat in social situations, such as at a restaurant or friend's house, increasing the risk of social isolation.

It's also important to note that there's no guarantee that this diet will reduce inflammation or disease-related symptoms in all people with autoimmune disorders.

However, those who experience a reduction in symptoms following this diet may be reticent to progress to the reintroduction phase, for fear it may bring the symptoms back.

This could become problematic, as remaining in the elimination phase can make it difficult to meet your daily nutrient requirements. Therefore, remaining in this phase for too long may increase your risk of developing nutrient deficiencies, as well as poor health over time.

This is why the reintroduction phase is crucial and should not be skipped.

If you're experiencing difficulties getting started with the reintroduction phase, consider reaching out to a registered dietitian or other medical professional knowledgeable about the AIP diet for personalized guidance.

Summary

The AIP diet may not work for everyone, and its elimination phase is very restrictive. This can make this diet isolating and hard to follow. It may also lead to a high risk of nutrient deficiencies if its reintroduction phase is avoided for too long.

Should You Try It?

The AIP diet is designed to help reduce inflammation, pain, or other symptoms caused by autoimmune diseases. As such, it may work best for people with autoimmune diseases, such as lupus, IBD, celiac disease, or rheumatoid arthritis.

Autoimmune diseases cannot be cured, but their symptoms may be managed. The AIP diet aims to help you do so by helping you identify which foods may be triggering your specific symptoms.

Evidence regarding the efficacy of this diet is currently limited to people with IBD and Hashimoto's disease.

However, based on the way in which this diet is believed to function, people with other autoimmune diseases may benefit from it, too.

There are currently few downsides to giving this diet a try, especially when performed under the supervision of a dietitian or other medical professional.

Seeking professional guidance prior to giving the AIP diet a try will help you better pinpoint which foods may be causing your specific symptoms, as well as ensure that you continue to meet your nutrient requirements as best as possible throughout all phases of this diet.

Summary

The AIP diet may reduce the severity of symptoms associated with various autoimmune diseases. However, it may be difficult to implement on your own, which is why guidance from a dietitian or medical professional is strongly recommended.

The bottom line

The AIP diet is an elimination diet designed to help reduce inflammation or other symptoms caused by autoimmune disorders.

It's comprised of two phases designed to help you identify and ultimately avoid the foods that may trigger inflammation and disease-specific symptoms. Research on its efficacy is limited but appears promising.

Due to its limited downsides, people with autoimmune disorders generally have little to lose by giving it a try. However, it's likely best to seek guidance from a qualified health professional to ensure you continue to meet your nutrient needs throughout all phases of this diet.

Aip Flatbread Recipe

Salads are a staple for an autoimmune diet, but sometimes you just want to have a piece of bread on the side. This AIP flatbread recipe is the perfect partner for your next salad night.

How To Make Bread For An Aip Diet

There are, of course, some obvious issues with eating bread on an autoimmune diet. Regular bread, whether white, whole wheat or you-name-it, is full of grains that will irritate your gut and trigger inflammation.

Even gluten-free and paleo bread and recipes can spell trouble for people following an AIP diet. Gluten-free bread can still contain sugar, and paleo bread are often made using nut flour, typically almond flour.

And they may be made with eggs, another food best avoided on AIP.

To address the egg situation, I "faked" an egg using gelatin. It's a good fit texture-wise for this recipe.

For the flour, I chose a mix of coconut and cassava flour. As it happens, many AIP, paleo, keto, and gluten-free baked goods work best with a combination of flour to achieve the right taste and texture.

Flavoring With Nutritional Yeast

Dairy, and therefore cheese, may be off-limits on your AIP diet, but there are some very viable alternatives.

Nutritional yeast, which are yellow-orange flakes often found in the bulk food section, happens to offer a nice cheesy flavor that works perfectly on this flatbread.

Ingredients

1.25 cups (140 g) coconut flour

1 cup (120 g) cassava flour

2 teaspoons (4 g) baking powder

1 Tablespoon (10 g) garlic powder

1 teaspoon mixed dried herbs (check the list of AIP herbs here)

A generous pinch salt

1 Tablespoon (8 g) Nutritional Yeast Flakes

1/2 cup (120 ml) boiling hot water

3 Tablespoons (18 g) gelatin powder

3 Tablespoons (45 ml) lukewarm water

3 Tablespoons (45 ml) hot water

2 Tablespoons (30 ml) olive oil

Sea salt flakes, to serve

Instructions

Preheat the oven to 350 F (175 C).

Combine the coconut flour, cassava flour, baking powder, garlic powder, dried herbs and salt in a large bowl. Set aside.

In a separate bowl, dissolve the nutritional yeast flakes in the boiling hot water and set aside.

Make a gelatin 'egg' by sprinkling the gelatin powder over the lukewarm water in a small bowl. Wait a minute or two, then add the hot water and stir well to dissolve. Add this dissolved gelatin mixture into the nutritional yeast water along with the olive oil. Whisk well.

Pour this wet mixture into the flour mixture and combine using a wooden spoon. It should come together as a dough – if it feels too dry, add 3-4 tablespoons of boiling hot water.

Divide the dough into 5 equal portions (approx. 3.5oz / 100g each) and use clean hands to shape into a flat ball. Press each portion (you may need to do this in two batches depending on the size of your tray) onto a large tray lined with parchment paper and compact down into a flat oval shape, just under ½-inch (1cm) thick. The dough can easily be manipulated, so smooth any edges that look as if they are 'cracking'.

Place in the oven for 12-15 minutes, rotating the tray halfway through. Remove and set aside to cool slightly. Scatter over sea salt flakes and enjoy!

Notes

All nutritional data are estimated and based on per serving amounts

Aip Waffles Recipe

What's in a Waffle?

This may be a first for you – actually making your waffle batter from scratch. Because let's be honest, most of you have that box of pancake mix hanging out in your pantry like a security blanket specially designed for breakfast emergencies.

Well, it's time to toss it out. Here's why. That cheerful cardboard box harbors a number of things you won't want to consume, including wheat flour, sugar, dextrose (another form of sugar), and sometimes soybean oil.

I know, it's so much easier to "just add water." But it's so not AIP.

Gelatin For Baking

Gelatin (I'm talking the unflavored stuff here) is a great thickening agent that can step in for eggs in many recipes. It's odorless and tasteless, a great flavor-neutral approach when you're just looking for a texture adjustment.

It will form a jelly when combined with water. It doesn't look delicious at this stage, but it helps you achieve that characteristic spongy waffle texture.

Prep Time: 5 minutes Cook Time: 10 minutes Yield: 2 servings 1x Category: Breakfast Cuisine: Belgian

Ingredients

2 teaspoons of gelatin (4 g)

2 Tablespoons of water (30 ml)

1 cup of cassava flour (120 g)

5 1/2 Tablespoons of coconut flour (39 g)

1/2 teaspoon of cream of tartar (2 g)

1/2 teaspoon of baking soda (2 g)

Pinch of salt

1 1/2 Tablespoons of coconut oil, solid weight, then melted (20 g)

2 Tablespoons of honey (30 ml), more to drizzle if desired

1/3 cup of hot water (79 ml)

Blueberries, to serve

Instructions

Put 2 tablespoons of hot water in a small bowl and sprinkle the gelatin over the water. Set aside.

Weigh out the solid coconut oil, then melt in a microwave.

Heat a greased waffle maker.

Combine the cassava flour, coconut flour, salt, cream of tartar, and baking soda in a bowl. Add the melted coconut oil, gelatin mixture, and honey to the bowl. Add the remaining hot water, stirring continuously. This will form a dough rather than the usual slurry consistency of waffles.

Add half the dough to the waffle maker and press down. Cook until crispy and holding its shape. Repeat for the second waffle.

Remove carefully and serve with a drizzle of honey and some blueberries, if desired.

Notes

All nutritional data are estimated and based on per serving amounts.

Aip Coconut Shrimp And Grits Recipe

A Twist on Grits

If you've never had the pleasure of eating traditional grits, I'm sorry. A savory corn-based dish, grits is often a breakfast item. The porridge-like dish is quite popular in the South.

Corn and grits by association are foods you want to stay away from for optimal health. They don't digest well and can cause or exacerbate gut issues. You can read my longer spiel on corn here.

I use coconut to create more digestible "grits." While the taste is different, they have a similar appearance and texture as normal grits. And the coconut pairs really well with the shrimp.

What Is Desiccated Coconut?

Quite simply, desiccated coconut is dried shredded coconut with a fancy name. It's a way for cooks and bakers who are in the know to show off their kitchen vocabulary and add texture and interest to their dishes.

Be very careful at the store when you're comparing labels. Desiccated coconut is sold in sweetened and unsweetened varieties. Make sure yours is unsweetened so you don't unknowingly derail your AIP diet efforts.

It's delicious toasted, but this recipe really isn't the place for that!

Prep Time: 10 minutes Cook Time: 15 minutes Yield: 4 servings 1x Category: Breakfast Cuisine: American

INGREDIENTS

2 Tablespoons (30 ml) olive oil, to cook with

15 button mushrooms, diced

2 cloves garlic, peeled and minced

9oz uncooked shrimp, peeled (255g)

generous squeeze lemon juice

1 cup (240 ml) coconut cream

2/3 cup unsweetened desiccated coconut

2 Tablespoons flat leaf parsley, diced (optional), for garnish

Crispy bacon bits (optional), for garnish

Salt to taste

Instructions

Add olive oil to a frying pan and sauté the mushrooms and garlic for 5 minutes.

Then add in the shrimp and cook until the shrimp turn pink. Add in lemon juice and season with salt. Set aside.

Make the coconut 'grits' by heating the desiccated coconut in the coconut cream.

Put the dish together by placing the mushroom shrimp mixture on top of the grits.

Garnish with parsley and bacon bits (optional).

Notes

All nutritional data are estimated and based on per serving amounts.

Blueberry Coconut Yogurt Smoothie Recipe [Paleo, Keto, Aip]

Blueberries are a delicious and nutritious berry to use on any diet. They're also delicious and full of antioxidants. That's why it's perfect for making smoothies with – it gives your smoothie a distinct flavor and lots of vitamins while only adding a small amount of sugar.

On a Paleo or AIP diet, it's easy to rely on bananas in your smoothies as the thickening agent. But this can make a very high sugar (and high carbohydrate) breakfast.

And if you're looking to lose weight or control your blood sugar, then it's best to avoid having quite that much sugar for breakfast.

So, try using coconut yogurt instead to make your smoothies thick and creamy. It's dairy-free, loaded with healthy probiotics, and delicious. Just make sure to buy one without added sugar.

Coconut yogurt is also perfect for those on a ketogenic diet as it adds in lots of healthy fats (and probiotics) into your diet without the extra carbs.

If you have trouble finding coconut yogurt at your local store, then you can make it yourself. Also, if you're on the autoimmune protocol, you'll probably want to make your own coconut yogurt to ensure all the ingredients are AIP-friendly. Here's a slow cooker recipe for making coconut yogurt. Here's a recipe that uses the Instant Pot. And here's one using a yogurt maker.

Blueberry Coconut Yogurt Smoothie Recipe

Step 1:

Place the coconut yogurt, coconut milk, blueberries, vanilla extract, and stevia into a blender. I think the vanilla extract and small amount of stevia as well as the blueberries provide plenty of sweetness to this smoothie. But if you find that you need more sweetness, then try adding a dash of raw honey as well.

Blueberry Coconut Yogurt Smoothie Recipe [Paleo, Keto,

Step 2:

Blend well and enjoy for a quick and delicious breakfast, brunch, or snack.

Blueberry Coconut Yogurt Smoothie Recipe [Paleo, Keto, A blueberry coconut yogurt smoothie recipe [paleo, keto, aip]

Prep Time: 5 minutes Cook Time: 0 minutes Yield: 2 servings 1x Category: Drinks Cuisine: American

Ingredients

1 pot (120 ml) of coconut yogurt

10 blueberries

1 cup coconut milk

1/2 teaspoon vanilla extract (omit for AIP)

Stevia to taste (omit for AIP)

Instructions

Place all the ingredients into the blender and blend really well.

Enjoy for a quick and nutritious breakfast or snack.

Notes

All nutritional data are estimated and based on per serving amounts.

Nutrition

Calories: 70Sugar: 2 gFat: 5 gCarbohydrates: 2 gFiber: 0 gProtein: 2 g

Paleo Passion Fruit Coconut Yogurt Parfait Recipe [Aip, Keto]

For those of us wanting to stay away from dairy on a Paleo diet, it can often mean giving up some easy breakfast favorites.

Yogurt is one of those dairy products that I often miss. I used to love eating Greek yogurt topped with fruits and nuts for a simple and delicious breakfast.

But luckily, coconut yogurt is a great dairy-free replacement.

Make your own Paleo coconut yogurt:

You can purchase coconut yogurt ready-made in many stores across North America and in Europe.

But if you're feeling up to it, you can also make it yourself. Take a look at this recipe if you want to give it a try. Or if you have an Instant Pot, then you can make coconut yogurt in that too.

What are passion fruits?

For this coconut yogurt parfait recipe, I used passionfruit to add a ton of delicious flavor, fragrance, and bring color.

So let me tell you a bit about this amazing fruit.

Passion fruit is often also known as passionfruit, granadilla, or maracuya. They're typically grown in tropical climates and are native to South America.

This delicious fruit is about the size of an egg but with a purple or dark red (or sometimes yellow) outer shell that can get quite brittle.

When you cut these fruits open, you'll find a bright yellow gel-like pulp with crunchy seeds that are edible. And if you smell them, you'll find an amazing tropical scent that reminds you of sandy white beaches.

How To Tell When Your Passion Fruit is Ripe?

In general, you can keep passion fruit at room temperature for quite a while. You'll find that the outer shell starts to get shriveled and wrinkled after a while. That's when they're ripe and ready to eat. If you eat them earlier, they might be a bit sour.

Paleo Passion Fruit Coconut Yogurt Parfait Recipe – Step-by-step Instructions

Step 1:

Slice your ripe passion fruit in half.

Step 2:

Spoon or pour your coconut yogurt into a small glass.

Step 3:

Get your other toppings (like the blueberries and nuts and seeds ready).

Step 4:

Put everything together. Scoop out the passion fruit with a spoon. Place 1 half into each glass on top of the coconut yogurt.

Step 5:

Top with the berries and crunchy nuts and seeds. Enjoy for a luxurious Paleo brunch or breakfast. Maybe impress your family or your guests with this beautiful dairy-free Paleo coconut yogurt parfait recipe next weekend!

Other Paleo Passion Fruit Recipes:

You can make a lot of other Paleo passion fruit recipes. They're very versatile and can add a gourmet touch to your meals.

Here are 2 other Paleo passion fruit recipes for you to try:

1. Paleo Passion Fruit Side Salad Recipe

Adding passionfruit to your salad adds crunch, natural sweetness, and flavor to your salad. You'll be sure to have guests asking what you did to make the typical boring side salad so exotic.

2. Paleo Strawberry Passionfruit Cooler Recipe

You can strain the passion fruit pulp to get the juice out. That juice can then be used to make delicious Paleo drinks like this strawberry passion fruit cooler.

Prep Time: 5 minutes Cook Time: 0 minutes Yield: 2 servings 1x Category: Dessert Cuisine: French

PRINT RECIPE

PIN RECIPE

INGREDIENTS

500 g coconut yogurt (if you buy it, make sure it doesn't have added sugar)

1 ripe passion fruit

2 heaped Tablespoons of nuts and seeds (I used a mixture of sesame seeds, pumpkin seeds, sunflower seeds, and goji berries) [Omit for AIP]

10 blueberries

INSTRUCTIONS

Divide the yogurt in half and place each half into a small wide glass (400 ml).

Cut open the passionfruit and spoon half onto the top of each yogurt parfait.

Add 1 heaped tablespoon of the nuts and seeds on top.

Add 5 blueberries to each glass.

Enjoy with a spoon.

NOTES

All nutritional data are estimated and based on per serving amounts.

Banana Pancakes Recipe [Aip, Paleo, Egg-Free]

It can be hard deciding what to eat for breakfast when you're on AIP (Paleo autoimmune protocol) and can't eat eggs or dairy products. So, if you're looking for a delicious AIP breakfast option (it's also Paleo-friendly of course), then give these AIP banana pancakes a try!

Paleo and AIP Banana Pancakes Recipe

Step 1:

Peel a ripe banana and place half of it into a mixing bowl.

Step 2:
Add the coconut flour to the mixing bowl.

Step 3:
Add in the baking soda, coconut oil, and honey/maple syrup.

Step 4:
Mix everything well to form a thick batter/dough.

Step 5:
Form golf-ball sized balls from the batter and press down to form a small pancake of around 1/4-inch (0.6 cm) thick. Place the

pancakes onto a baking tray lined with parchment paper.

Step 6:
Bake for 20 minutes in the oven, remove and then let cool for a bit before enjoying. Serve with extra honey or maple syrup if you want it.

Prep Time: 10 minutes Cook Time: 20 minutes Yield: 2 servings 1x Category: Breakfast Cuisine: American

Ingredients

1/2 bananas mashed

1/4 cup (28 g) coconut flour

1/8 teaspoon (0.5 g) baking soda

1 Tablespoon (15 ml) coconut oil

1 Tablespoon (15 ml) raw honey or maple syrup

1 Tablespoon (7 g) gelatin

3 Tablespoons (45 ml) hot water

Extra raw honey or maple syrup for serving

Instructions

Preheat oven to 300 F (150 C).

Place the mashed bananas, coconut flour, baking soda, coconut oil, and honey/ maple syrup into a mixing bowl. Dissolve the gelatin in the hot water and then add into the mixing bowl as well.

Mix well to form a batter.

Make the batter into around a golf-ball size and press down to a pancake of around 1/4-inch (0.6 cm) thick. Batter should make 4 pancakes.

Bake for 20 minutes and remove carefully from oven. Cool a little and then eat. Drizzle with extra honey or maple syrup if desired.

Sweet Potato Breakfast Hash Recipe [Paleo, Aip, Gluten-Free]

This breakfast recipe is a fantastic way to use any leftover meats from the night before. It's also a great opportunity to add in your favorite herbs. I used leftover beef when I made this, but it would work with leftover turkey, chicken, or ham. So, remember this recipe for the morning after Christmas dinner!

This recipe is pretty easy to make – the sweet potato and zucchini add a sweet touch to the dish, and adding in your favorite herbs will enable you to customize this recipe to suit your tastes (as well as what you have handy). I used fresh thyme when I made it, but rosemary, cilantro, basil, and parsley.

STEP 1: Chop your veggies.

STEP 2: Shred the sweet potatoes and zucchini using the shredding attachment of your food processor (or use a grater).

STEP 3: Place coconut oil into the saute pan (or skillet) and then add in the shredded sweet potatoes and zucchini. Saute until they soften.

STEP 4: Next, add in the leftover meat.

STEP 5: Add in your favorite herbs.

STEP 6: Saute until the sweet potato is tender. Then serve.

Prep Time: 10 minutes Cook Time: 5 minutes Yield: 2 servings 1x
Category: Breakfast Cuisine: American

Ingredients

1 sweet potato, shredded

1/2 zucchini, shredded

1 cup leftover meat, shredded (approx. 6 oz)

1 Tablespoon (2 g) fresh thyme leaves, finely chopped (or use 1 tsp
(1 g) dried thyme or use other herbs of your choosing)

1 Tablespoons (15 ml) coconut oil for cooking

Salt to taste

Instructions

Place 1 Tablespoon of coconut oil into a frying pan on medium
heat.

Add in the shredded sweet potato, shredded zucchini, and left
over meat. Cook until the sweet potato starts to get tender
(approx. 5 minutes).

Add in the herbs and salt to taste

Lemon Fried Avocado Recipe [Paleo, Aip]

I was frying some eggs one day and pondering what to eat with my fried eggs when I saw some avocados in our fruit bowl.

I'd once come across a recipe for grilled avocados, so somehow my brain connected some dots and went:

Why not fry some avocado slices in coconut oil!

Lemon Fried Avocado Paleo Recipe

So, I halved an avocado, removed the stone, and scored inside the avocado to cut it into slices. I suggest picking an avocado that isn't too ripe (not mushy) but also not too hard (i.e., you can cut into it without too much trouble).

lemon fried avocado recipe paleo aip

Then I put the avocado slices into the frying pan with the coconut oil I was already frying my eggs with.

Fry the avocado slices (turning them gently) until slightly browned on all sides.

lemon fried avocado recipe paleo aip

Squeeze a bit of lemon juice on top and sprinkle salt on top (use lemon salt for some extra deliciousness). I made some lemon fried avocado recently and served them with some sashimi.

Lemon Fried Avocado Recipe Aip Paleo Keto

lemon fried avocado recipe paleo aip

lemon fried avocado recipe [paleo, aip]

Prep Time: 2 minutes Cook Time: 5 minutes Yield: 2 servings 1x Category: Appetizer, Side dish Cuisine: American

INGREDIENTS

1 ripe avocado (not too soft), cut into slices

1 Tablespoon coconut oil

1 Tablespoon lemon juice

Salt to taste (or lemon salt)

INSTRUCTIONS

Add the coconut oil to a frying pan. Place the avocado slices into the oil gently.

Fry the avocado slices (turning gently) so that all sides are slightly browned.

Sprinkle the lemon juice and salt over the slices and serve warm.

Aip Chicken Lettuce Wraps Recipe

This AIP chicken lettuce wraps recipe is a light, refreshing meal that's perfect for a hot summer day. It's so easy to whip up you can make it after work!

Lettuce Wraps Around The World

Lettuce wraps have gained in popularity in the U.S. in recent times thanks to the popularity of low-carb diets. In other parts of the world, however, lettuce wraps are old news.

Lettuce wraps are common throughout Asia and Thailand. In Thai cuisine, the meat in lettuce wraps is often flavored with fish sauce and/or tamarind paste.

In this recipe, I use coconut aminos to replicate the traditional flavor of chicken wraps without cheating your autoimmune diet. Ginger also adds to the taste of Thailand in these wraps.

Picking Your Lettuce

Believe it or not, there is an art and a bit of luck involved in selecting the best lettuce for your wraps. Too firm, and they'll crack. Too weak, and they'll fall apart.

Iceberg lettuce is nice and firm, which helps the wraps to hold their form. Butter works really nicely as a soft option.

Bibb is another viable option, as is romaine. You may have to work with what is available.

Regardless of what kind of lettuce you go with, pick a good specimen without obvious wilting or holes.

More AIP Lunch Ideas

I really like making these lettuce wraps for lunch in the summer. If you need even more ideas for eating lunch on your autoimmune diet, check these out.

Prep Time: 10 minutes Cook Time: 10 minutes Yield: 2 servings 1x Category: Dinner Cuisine: American

Ingredients

2 Tablespoons (30 ml) avocado oil

2 oz mushrooms, finely chopped (60g)

2 cloves of garlic, peeled and minced

1 small piece ginger, peeled and minced

9 oz ground chicken (255 g)

1 teaspoon (5 ml) lemon juice

2 Tablespoons (30 ml) coconut aminos

4 large iceberg lettuce leaves

1 spring onion, finely sliced

cilantro, to garnish

Instructions

Heat the avocado oil in a pan and cook the mushrooms until caramelized.

Add the garlic, ginger, and ground chicken and cook until the chicken has cooked thoroughly, stirring regularly. Stir in the lemon juice and coconut aminos and remove the pan from the heat.

Spoon the mixture into large, open lettuce leaves and scatter over the spring onions and cilantro. Wrap the leaves in on themselves and enjoy!

Notes

All nutritional data are estimated and based on per serving amounts.

Nutrition

Calories: 303Sugar: 1 gFat: 23 gCarbohydrates: 3 gFiber: 0 gProtein: 20 g

Aip Waldorf Salad

If you eat the same salad every day, it's easy to become bored. Fortunately, this AIP waldorf salad offers an amazingly unconventional lunch or dinner option.

Perhaps the signature feature of a traditional waldorf salad is its mayonnaise base. To make this version AIP-friendly, I created a homemade dressing that pairs nicely with apples, celery, and grapes.

Coconut Dressing

It's waldorf gone tropical! This special dressing is made by combining coconut cream with lemon juice.

This combination may curdle on you at first, but if you're bothered by that possibility go ahead and make a larger batch and emulsify it with a hand blender.

Lactose intolerant or just generally dairy-free folks are already wise to using coconut milk to make safe salad dressings. Now you can too!

Coconut Milk

You'll get the coconut cream required for this recipe by taking it off the top of a container of coconut milk. If you're not well versed in shopping for coconut milk, here are a few tips:

Look for BPA-free cans. A lot of coconut milk can be found in cans containing BPA, which has been linked to adverse health effects. Fortunately, there are BPA-free options.

Look for a short ingredient list. Stick to an option that only contains coconut and water.

Look out for added sweeteners. An unsweetened variety will still contain naturally occurring sugar, and it's plenty sweet enough.

This AIP waldorf salad omits walnuts, but you can add some toasted desiccated coconut on top.

Prep Time: 10 minutes Cook Time: 0 minutes Yield: 1 serving 1x Category: Appetizer Cuisine: American

PRINT RECIPE

PIN RECIPE

INGREDIENTS

2 Tablespoons coconut cream (30 ml) (from the top of a can of re-

frigerated coconut milk)

1 teaspoon (5 ml) lemon juice

Salt to taste

1 Granny Smith or another green apple, thinly sliced

1 stalk of celery, thinly sliced at an angle

10 grapes, halved

1 head of romaine lettuce, chopped

Instructions

Make the AIP salad dressing by combining coconut cream and lemon juice. Season with salt to taste.

Add the dressing to all the remaining ingredients and toss until evenly coated.

NOTES

All nutritional data are estimated and based on per serving amounts.

Nutrition

Calories: 141Sugar: 19 gFat: 5 gCarbohydrates: 26 gFiber: 5 gProtein: 0 g

Grass-fed beef burgers are not only AIP, Paleo, and Keto, but they're also just really tasty and easy to make.

So, whip these up no matter what diet you're on. You can also switch out the seasonings or add in some vegetables to change the flavors.

Here are some different seasoning options for AIP burgers:

Thai Burgers – Chopped fresh basil leaves with a dash of coconut aminos

Onion Burgers – Finely chopped green onions with onion powder

Garlic Burgers – Finely chopped onions with garlic powder

Veggie Burgers – Finely chopped asparagus, spinach, and green onions

Test them out and see which one is your favorite. Personally, I find the onions with garlic are delicious every time!

Aip Italian Burgers Recipe

For the AIP Italian burgers, I used Italian seasoning with some garlic and onion powder for a super fast and easy mixture. Then just form burger patties and grill. Or if it's too wet or cold to grill, then you can also pan-fry these in some coconut oil.

What To Serve With

Serve these AIP burgers with salads and a bacon veggie saute for a complete AIP meal. Or grill some asparagus and mushrooms as a quick side dish. Season with sea salt when you're eating.

Prep Time: 5 minutes Cook Time: 10 minutes Yield: 2 servings 1x Category: Lunch, Dinner Cuisine: Italian

Ingredients

1 lb of grass-fed ground beef (450 g)

2 Tablespoons of Italian seasoning (6 g)

2 Tablespoons of garlic powder (20 g)

1 Tablespoon of onion powder (7 g)

INSTRUCTIONS

Mix all the ingredients together well and form burger patties from the mixture.

Grill or pan-fry in coconut oil until done to your liking.

Notes

All nutritional data are estimated and based on per serving amounts.

Nutrition

Calories: 640Sugar: 3 gFat: 48 gCarbohydrates: 9 gFiber: 1 gProtein: 39 g

Smoked Salmon And Cucumber Ham Wraps Recipe [Paleo, Keto, Aip]

If you're looking for an easy lunch that's delicious and nutritious, then try these smoked salmon and cucumber ham wraps. It's perfect regardless of whether you're on a Paleo, Ketogenic, or AIP diet.

These wraps take just 5 minutes to put together so you can also make these for an egg-free breakfast or brunch or as a quick snack.

Instructions For Making Smoked Salmon and Cucumber Ham Wraps

Step 1:
Prepare a spinach salad to serve the wraps with. You can use any green leafy salad you wish.

Step 2:
Create thin cucumber slices by cutting a cucumber in half and then use a potato peeler to create thin slices.

Step 3:
Typically cream cheese goes well with smoked salmon, but for a dairy-free and AIP (autoimmune protocol) version, I've used coconut cream instead. Another option if you're not AIP is to use Paleo mayo instead. However, I really enjoyed the coconut flavor the coconut cream gave to the dish.

Step 4:
Place a slice of ham on a plate and spread the coconut cream on the ham. If you can't find ham that's suitable for AIP, then you can also use lettuce as the wrap.

Step 5:

Place the slices of smoked salmon on top of the ham slice. If you're using thin slices of ham, then you might need to use several slices so it doesn't break when the wrap is created.

Step 6:
Place several cucumber slices on top of the salmon.

Step 7:
Roll everything up.

Prep Time: 5 minutes Cook Time: 0 minutes Yield: 2 servings 1x Category: Breakfast, Snack Cuisine: American

INGREDIENTS

4 slices of ham

1/2 cucumber, cut into thin slices

3.5 oz (100 g) smoked salmon

1 Tablespoon (15 ml) coconut cream

Green salad to serve with

INSTRUCTIONS

Spread coconut cream on each slice of ham.

Place smoked salmon slices on top of each slice of ham.

Place the thin cucumber slices on top.

Roll the wrap up and place on top of the green salad to serve.

NUTRITION

Serving Size: 2 wrapsCalories: 210Sugar: 0 gFat: 10 gCarbohy-drates: 0 gFiber: 0 gProtein: 29 g

Aip Avocado Salad Recipe

Salads can get boring for even the most veg-loving herbivores, but the food restrictions on AIP take things to a whole other level. This lettuce-free AIP avocado salad recipe is a fresh new take on lunch.

An Ingredient That Can't Be Beet

See what I did there? Most people love avocado, and I'll bet you do too if you're diving into this recipe.

But there's another underrated ingredient that's worthy of your attention, especially if you're following autoimmune protocol.

I included beets in this salad as a colorful counterpart to the avocado. In addition to presenting a pleasing picture, beets contain different nutrients so you'll benefit from the overall well-roundedness of your plate.

Beets get their rich red color from a pigment known as betalain. They also give you some of nature's necessities, like folate, manganese, vitamin C, iron, and potassium.

Athletes have been known to drink beet juice to enhance performance. If it works for the pros, imagine what it could do for average folks!

The Main Event: Avocado

There are a couple of things you can do to make sure this AIP avocado salad is in prime condition.

First, pick a ripe avocado. The right candidate should be dark green and should yield to pressure without being squishy or soft.

Indentations could be a sign of bruising; avoid avocados that have significant bumps.

At home, you'll need to peel the avocado. I like to cut mine in wedges before pulling the peel away.

Squeeze a bit of lemon juice over the sliced avocado to keep it from turning brown (not a good look).

Add the other ingredients, and your salad should be perfection!

The Authority on AIP

Starting any diet can be overwhelming, but autoimmune protocol takes things to a whole new level.

While you have to be more careful than many other diets, it can have a profound impact on your health.

Take a detailed look at what AIP entails and the conditions it may help in this free guide. You'll learn what not to eat, find answers to common questions, and discover more great recipes like this avocado salad.

Description

A simple salad of creamy avocado, earthy beets, and pickled red onions.

Ingredients

1/4 red onion (28 g), thinly sliced

1 Tablespoon (15 ml) of red wine vinegar

1 large avocado (200 g), peeled and sliced

squeeze lemon juice

salt

1 small cooked, pickled beetroot (82 g), sliced

1 small carrot (50 g), peeled and sliced into matchsticks

olive oil, to drizzle

chopped chives, to garnish

Instructions

Place the red onions and red wine vinegar in a small bowl and leave to pickle while you prepare the rest of the salad.

Season the diced avocado with salt and squeeze the lemon juice over top.

Divide the avocado, beets, and carrots onto two plates and drizzle each with a little olive oil. Divide the pickled red onions between the two salads and drizzle over any remaining vinegar. Garnish with chives and serve.

Notes

All nutritional data are estimated and based on per serving amounts.

Nutrition

Calories: 200Sugar: 6 gFat: 15 gCarbohydrates: 18 gFiber: 8 gProtein: 3 g

Aip Bacon-Wrapped Salmon Recipe

This AIP bacon-wrapped salmon recipe is a match made in heaven. It's a luxurious low-carb date night kind of meal you can make in a jiffy.

The History Of Salmon As A Food Source

People have been dining on this delicious fatty fish off the coast of Europe since Palaeolithic times. Native Americans ate a salmon-rich diet, and European settlers also took to eating the fish.

There was a time when salmon was prevalent in both the Atlantic and Pacific coasts, but the advent of modern canning and food preservation methods led to overfishing and created scarcity.

Today, the majority of commercial salmon is produced at salmon farms.

What Sets This Salmon Apart

There are a few things I love about this particular autoimmune protocol diet recipe. The delicious smoked bacon adds loads of flavor to the fish. It is unlikely you'll need extra seasoning, but have some sea salt flakes on the ready just in case it's not to your liking.

Chopped tarragon also makes this salmon special. If you don't use it a lot, tarragon is bittersweet, with a distinctive flavor. Some tasters detect hints of licorice and vanilla in the spice.

Use a conservative amount of tarragon if you've never had it. If you like it you can always add more.

Prep Time: 10 minutes Cook Time: 20 minutes Yield: 2 servings 1x
Category: Dinner Cuisine: American

Ingredients

2 filets of salmon, fresh or frozen (340 g)

4 slices of bacon (112 g)

1 Tablespoon of olive oil (15 ml)

2 Tablespoons of tarragon (32 g), to garnish

Lemon wedges, to serve

Instructions

Preheat the oven to 350°F (180°C).

Pat the salmon fillets dry. Wrap bacon around the fillets.

Place fillets onto a roasting tray and drizzle with the olive oil. Bake
for 15-20 minutes.

Serve garnished with chopped tarragon and lemon wedges.

NOTES

All nutritional data are estimated and based on per serving
amounts.

Nutrition

Calories: 776Sugar: 0 gFat: 63 gCarbohydrates: 0 gFiber: 0
gProtein: 48 g

Aip Baked Lemon Salmon Recipe

Easy peasy lemon squeazy. This AIP baked lemon salmon recipe may be simple, but it is an amazing dinner option for your auto-immune diet.

Most people don't chomp on lemons the way you might eat other citrus fruits, such as oranges or grapefruit. That doesn't mean they don't have a place in your AIP diet, however. They work really well in a lot of recipes.

How to Buy the Best Lemons

Lemons, lemon juice, and lemon zest are great tools to have in your AIP cooking toolbox, as they offer a healthy way to introduce flavor into many dishes.

When you're shopping for lemons, select candidates that feel heavy in comparison to their peers. The fruit should give readily if given a gentle squeeze – a thinner rind usually means there is more juice inside, which is desirable.

Visually, the lemon should be bright yellow and shiny. Avoid fruit with greenish areas, as that indicates it's not ripe yet. You'll also want to stay away from lemons with blemishes or oddly wrinkled skin.

Aip Fish Recipes

While I like salmon, and it's a great source of healthy fats, I understand that it's not to everyone's taste. Here are some additional AIP fish recipes you can use to increase your intake of fish.

Prep Time: 5 minutes Cook Time: 20 minutes Yield: 2 servings 1x Category: Dinner Cuisine: American

Ingredients

2 Lemons (60 ml), sliced thinly

2 Filets of salmon, fresh or frozen (340 g)

2 Tablespoons of olive oil (30 ml)

Salt and freshly ground black pepper

Thyme sprigs, to garnish

Beetroot salad, to serve

INSTRUCTIONS

Preheat the oven to 350°F (180°C).

Divide the lemon slices in half. Take one half of the lemons and place on a sheet of foil. Put the salmon on top of the lemons and cover with the second half. Drizzle olive oil over the fillets.

Fold the foil over the fillets, sealing completely. Bake in the oven for 20 minutes.

Season the salmon with salt and serve garnished with thyme alongside a fresh green beetroot salad.

Notes

All nutritional data are estimated and based on per serving amounts.

Nutrition

Calories: 571Sugar: 2 gFat: 44 gCarbohydrates: 2 gFiber: 0 gProtein: 42 g

Aip Shrimp Fried Rice

On an AIP diet, you learn to fall back in love with seafood (because seafood is really nutritious plus delicious). This AIP shrimp fried rice dish is so fresh and flavorful you'll never miss takeout again!

Adapting for an Autoimmune Diet

Traditional shrimp fried rice is actually not too far off from our version. Only the rice and cooking oil are modified to keep you healthy and happy.

For the rice, you'll be using cauliflower, the old standby. Chop it in your food processor, and make sure you get the water out – nobody likes soggy "rice"!

For the cooking oil, I suggest using avocado oil. It's got a very light flavor so it won't overpower the shrimp or combine badly with the coconut aminos.

Benefits Of Avocado Oil

I use avocado oil in place of some less virtuous cooking oils for a lot of reasons. First, it's a pretty healthy fat.

Avocado oil features oleic acid, which helps manage glucose levels, reduces blood pressure, and may even help burn fat.

Also, avocado oil has a high smoke point, which makes it a good choice for searing, roasting, grilling, or pan frying. It's used to pan fry the shrimp and cook the veggies in this meal.

Prep Time: 10 minutes Cook Time: 15 minutes Yield: 2 servings 1x
Category: Lunch, Dinner Cuisine: Chinese

PRINT RECIPE

PIN RECIPE

Ingredients

0.5 lb of shrimp (225 g), peeled

1 medium onion (110 g), diced

2 cloves of garlic (6 g), diced

1 head of cauliflower (600 g), broken into florets

2 carrots (100 g), diced

2 green onions (10 g), diced

4 Tablespoons of avocado oil (60 ml), to cook in

2 Tablespoons of coconut aminos (30 ml)

Salt, to taste

Instructions

Add avocado oil to a frying pan and cook the peeled shrimp along with the diced onion and garlic until the shrimp is cooked and the onions are slightly browned. Remove from the pan and set aside.

Food process the cauliflower florets in a food processor until it forms rice-like small pieces.

Make sure to dry the cauliflower before food processing and squeeze out excess water after.

Add the cauliflower rice and carrots to the pan and cook until softened.

Add back the shrimp, onion, garlic and then top with green onions. Season with coconut aminos and salt to taste.

Notes

All nutritional data are estimated and based on per serving amounts.

Nutrition

Calories: 482Sugar: 12 gFat: 31 gCarbohydrates: 27 gFiber: 9 gProtein: 29 g